Mileidys López Bacallao
Dailyn López Santana
Alicia García Pérez

Psychotropic drugs in older adults

Mileidys López Bacallao
Dailyn López Santana
Alicia García Pérez

Psychotropic drugs in older adults

Proposed actions to reduce consumption

ScienciaScripts

Imprint

Any brand names and product names mentioned in this book are subject to trademark, brand or patent protection and are trademarks or registered trademarks of their respective holders. The use of brand names, product names, common names, trade names, product descriptions etc. even without a particular marking in this work is in no way to be construed to mean that such names may be regarded as unrestricted in respect of trademark and brand protection legislation and could thus be used by anyone.

Cover image: www.ingimage.com

This book is a translation from the original published under ISBN 978-620-2-15062-0.

Publisher:
Sciencia Scripts
is a trademark of
Dodo Books Indian Ocean Ltd. and OmniScriptum S.R.L publishing group

120 High Road, East Finchley, London, N2 9ED, United Kingdom
Str. Armeneasca 28/1, office 1, Chisinau MD-2012, Republic of Moldova, Europe
Printed at: see last page
ISBN: 978-620-7-31173-6

TITLE:

PSYCHOTROPIC DRUGS IN OLDER ADULTS
PROPOSAL OF ACTIONS TO REDUCE THE CONSUMPTION OF PSYCHOTROPIC DRUGS

Authors:

Mileidys López Bacallao MSc.

Degree in Pharmacy. Master's Degree in Natural Medicines Development. Assistant Professor at UCMVC

Dr. Dailyn López Santana.

Doctor of Medicine. Specialist of I degree in MGI

Dr. Alicia García Pérez.

Doctor in Medicine. Specialist of I degree in MGI and Geriatrics. Assistant Professor at UCMVC

SUMMARY

Older adults are targets of polypharmacy and inappropriate prescription, and self-medication with psychoactive substances is a potential risk for them. With the aim of proposing actions focused on reducing the consumption of psychotropic drugs in older adults of the Medical Clinic 21, a descriptive, cross-sectional study was conducted in 2021. Through an interview and a documentary review guide, information was obtained from 53 older adults selected by criteria for the study. It was found that 79.2% belonged to the female sex, 24.5% had primary schooling, 64.1% reported always using psychotropic drugs, 71.7% consumed the drug that appeared, 75.5% used more than one. The use of hypnotics was predominant in 64.2% of the women and 15.1% of the men. The 64.2% acquired the drugs without prescription. Sleep disorders were reported as the cause by 52.8% of the patients, 79.2% denied the occurrence of adverse events. 66.1% were unaware of the risks of the use of psychotropic drugs in the elderly. A proposal of actions was designed to increase the knowledge of the elderly about the risks of these drugs and to promote intersectoriality for the realization of entertainment activities that allow them to leave the daily routine, relax and avoid stress and practice other alternatives that reduce the consumption of psychotropic drugs.

CONTENTS

INTRODUCTION

Throughout the life cycle, aging is a phenomenon present from the very process of conception until death, which causes a set of physiological modifications as a consequence of the action of time on living beings.[1]

The aging of populations, although heterogeneous, is an inescapable fact that is occurring in all countries. As the fertility rate decreases and life expectancy increases, the proportion of people aged 60 and over should increase in all regions of the planet. It is known that the number of individuals in the world over the age of 60 has risen, with a forecast of more than 1.2 billion by 2025, i.e., it will grow annually at a rate of 2.5% compared to the total world population, which is growing by only 1.7%.[2]

In the region of the Americas, the process is developing with different characteristics. There are countries in each of the stages of the demographic transition; some, such as Bolivia, Guatemala and Haiti, have an incipient aging population, while others, such as Uruguay, Argentina, Barbados and Cuba, have advanced aging. Heterogeneity is not only demographic, but also economic, social and cultural.[2,3] Cuba, in 2000, had 64 older adults for every 100 children. In 2050 this ratio will be one of the highest in the world with 220 older adults for every 100 children.[4] Among the provinces with the highest aging we have: the western (excluding Pinar del Río) and central provinces, and a lower aging in the eastern provinces, related to the fertility and mortality levels of the territories.[5] Villa Clara is the most aged province in the country; in 2021, 25% of its population was 60 years old or older. [6]

During the process of senescence, physiological changes occur that lead to a lower functional reserve and a decrease in the capacity to adapt to these changes. This means that in the elderly, the response of the organism to the alterations caused by a disease or the administration of any drug is different from that of the young organism; and therefore, the effectiveness of pharmacotherapy could be affected.[7]

As the age of the individual advances, morbidity increases and the prevalence of chronic diseases and disabilities are higher than in other stages of life, leading to an increase in the use of healthcare resources and a higher consumption of drugs by the elderly compared to the rest of the population.[5,7]

According to a study conducted in the largest of the Antilles, the elderly have a high consumption profile, especially after the age of 65. Eighty-one percent of them take medications and two thirds of them take more than one drug on a regular basis. Thirty percent of people over 75 years of age take more than three drugs.[8] Psychotropic drugs, together with antibiotics and analgesics, are precisely the three pharmacological groups most consumed by this population segment in Cuba.[9] Similarly, other research corroborates that worldwide the consumption of psychotropic drugs in the elderly has increased in the last 20 years, with a prevalence ranging between 14 and 38%.[10, 11, 12] Faced with this situation, society faces a major challenge, both from an economic and ethical point of view.

The origin of this increased risk is multifactorial: older adults also present a high prevalence of polypathology, polypharmacy and potentially inappropriate prescribing and a series of physiological changes that determine alterations in the pharmacokinetic processes of many frequently prescribed drugs.[10]

Self-medication and polypharmacy are the main patterns of medication consumption within the irrational use of drugs. Both practices have become a worldwide health problem and constitute a potential risk for the subjects who practice them. In the daily work in the clinics, there are patients who live alone, retired, without family support or new life projects. All these factors lead patients to feel sad, anguished, discouraged and depressed, so that the consumption of psychotropic drugs is increasing at alarming rates, constituting a serious concern for the health area, making it necessary to establish psychoeducational strategies that collaborate in their solution and allow eradicating or attenuating this health problem.

Precisely in the municipality of Santo Domingo in the province of Villa Clara, where population aging is one of the most important challenges to be assumed by the public health system and particularly in the locality of Rodrigo, which shows 22.4% of older adults,[13] the consumption of psychotropic drugs by this age group is high. Taking this into account, it was decided to carry out the present research since by emphasizing the educational aspect we will be able to achieve greater cooperation.

Problem statement:

How to contribute to reduce the consumption of psychotropic drugs in older adults of the Medical Clinic N° 21 of Rodrigo, belonging to the Policlínico Docente Manuel Piti Fajardo of Santo Domingo in the period 2020-2022?

Objectives:

GENERAL:

1- To propose a system of actions to reduce the consumption of psychotropic drugs in older adults of the Family Medical Clinic N° 21 in the town of Rodrigo.

SPECIFIC:

1- To distribute the sample according to sociodemographic variables of interest by sex.

2- Describe the sample according to forms of psychotropic drug use and routes of acquisition.

3- To determine the reason for consumption according to sex.

4- Describe the occurrence of adverse drug events.

5- To identify the knowledge of older adults about the risks of psychotropic drug use in the elderly.

6- To design actions that promote a decrease in the consumption of psychotropic drugs in the older adults studied.

THEORETICAL FRAMEWORK

General information on aging.

Aging is the set of inevitable and irreversible modifications that occur in living beings over the years. It is a lifelong process and its effects vary according to the individual, with old age being considered to begin at the age of 60.[14]

From the beginning of human history until the beginning of the 20th century, human beings achieved an average lifespan of 47 years, but from then until today, this average has increased by almost 30 years. In this century, the planet is expected to quadruple its elderly population in the next fifty years.[15]

At present, it is estimated that there are around 901 million elderly people on the planet, representing 12% of the global population, and it is estimated that by 2050 this will rise to 2100 million, or 21.5%. Currently, one in ten people is over 60 years of age, but by 2050 this proportion will increase to one in five.[2,15]

In Spain, life expectancy is 80 years for women and 74 years for men. In the United States the geriatric population has grown dramatically, the number of people over 65 years of age has increased from 4% in 1900.[16]

The aging of Latin America and the Caribbean has been very rapid and will become more so. In 2000, according to data from the Economic Commission for Latin America and the Caribbean (ECLAC), there were slightly more than 41,000,000 elderly people in the region, and it is estimated that by 2025 there will be twice as many, or 98,000,000. Within this group, those over 80 will increase much faster, at a growth rate of 4% per year, which occurs in poor populations and accentuates heterogeneity and inequalities, especially socioeconomic and gender inequalities.

There are 11 238 661 inhabitants in Cuba, 19.4% of whom are over 60 years of age, and life expectancy at birth is 78.45 years. Currently in the country, it is women who enjoy the highest survival rates, reaching a life expectancy of 80.45 years compared to 76.50 years for men, thus evidencing the phenomenon 17,18,19 known as the feminization of aging. ''

Epidemiology on medication use in the elderly.

At present, the development of science and technology have conditioned the emergence of drugs as an instrument of health care. The sale of these drugs in the world exceeds 380 billion dollars a year. Over the last 30 years, the profitability of the pharmaceutical industry has grown faster than any other industry. Around 30 percent of health resources are destined to this area; however, there is evidence of the inadequate use of these. It is pointed out that 50% of the drugs that are sold, prescribed, dispensed or consumed are used inappropriately.[20]

Medicines are the most widely used medical technology in the contemporary world; they have saved lives and prevented diseases, but their indiscriminate use has turned them into a public health problem.[7,20]

U.S. data show that 30% of all prescriptions are made by the elderly, a particularly striking figure when considering that the elderly represent only 15-18% of the total population. This high rate of use has also been documented in other countries such as Canada and the U.K. In addition to formal prescriptions, 40% of them regularly use at least one over-the-counter drug, which are often not reported in regular medical records.[21] In Spain, between 75.6 and 96% of the elderly population receive 1 or more drugs, with an average of between 4.2 and 8 drugs per person per day. Those prescribed by the family physician, by various specialists and self-medication add up to a significant number of preparations that the patient takes on a more or less regular basis. Among these there can be duplications and side effects can occur, with signs and symptoms that complicate the diagnostic process.[22,23]

In Cuba, the production of medicines is in the hands of the state. The industry works in coordination with the National Health System and produces and distributes medicines according to the country's epidemiological picture. An educational strategy is developed through the use of television to promote the rational use of medicines, with special emphasis on increasing therapeutic compliance and reducing self-medication. In addition, almost all medicines are dispensed by prescription and the rest are acquired through the control card system according to the dosage prescribed for the month.[24]

Research has shown that drug consumption in the Cuban population increases with age in number and quantity, with 1.6 drugs per person. Older adults have a high consumption profile, especially after the age of 65, with higher consumption among women. [8,25]

Western society faces an important challenge, both from an economic and ethical point of view, in relation to their appropriate use, especially those with psychoactive effects, since these are the ones that have experienced the greatest increase in their use in the elderly in recent years. [26]

Psychotropic drugs. Concept and classification.

The term psychopharmaceutical comes from the Greek, pysche: mind, tropera: to turn. They are drugs that act on the Central Nervous System modifying the behavior of individuals, alleviating the symptomatology of mental disorders and favoring psychological and mental readjustment. [10, 27]

Their classification is summarized below: [28]

- Anxiolytics and sedatives:

1- Benzodiazepines:

    a) Potent: clonazepam and alprazolam.

    b) Medium potency: diazepam, chlorodiazepoxide, lorazepam and midazolam.

    c) Low potency: oxazepam

2- No benzodiazepines:

    a) Azapirones: 5 HT1A receptor agonists: buspirone (poor sedative effect)

    b) Cyclopyrrolones: zoplicone and suriclone

    c) Imidazopyridines: zolpidem and alpidem

    d) Beta-carbolines (abecarnil)

    e) Beta antagonists

    f) Miscellaneous agents: paraldehyde, chloral hydrate, and sedative antihistamines (diphenhydramine).

<u>- Hypnotics:</u>

a) Benzodiazepines: brotizolam, loprazolam, triazolam, midazolam, flunitrazepam, flurazepam.

b) Cyclopyrrolones: zopiclone

c) Imidazopyridines: zolpidem, and pyrazolopyrimidines: zaleplon

<u>- Antidepressants:</u>

1- Class I: monoamine oxidase inhibitors (MAOIs)

a) Non-selective (MAO-A and MAO-B): phenelzine, isocarboxazid

b) Selective:

-MAO-A: chlorgiline, mocoblemide

-MAO-B: selegiline and almoxatone

2- Class II: pure neuronal receptor blockers:

a) IIA: noradrenergics and serotonergics

- Tricyclic antidepressants (TCAs): imipramine, amitriptyline, clomipramine, desipramine, nortriptyline

b) IIB: relatively selective, atypical:

- Of the serotonergic neuron (SSRI): fluoxetine, paroxetine and sertraline.

- Of the noradrenergic neuron (NARI): reboxetine, maprotiline

- From the dopaminergic neuron: amineptin

c) IIC: noradrenergic and serotonergic (IRNS):

- New antidepressants: venlafaxine and duloxetine

d) IID: noradrenergic and dopaminergic:

-Atypical antidepressants: bupropion

3- Class III: drugs with a mechanism of action different from those of class I and II:

a) IIIA: noradrenergic and dopaminergic modulators (amoxapine).

b) IIIB: noradrenergic modulators (mianserin)

c) IIICs: serotonergic modulators (tianeptine, trazodone, nefazodone)

d) IIID: noradrenergic and serotonergic modulators (NASSAs): mirtazapine

<u>- Antipsychotics:</u>

1- Typical:

a) Phenothiazine derivatives: Chlorpromazine, Thioridazine, Levomepromazine, Trifluoperazine, Fluphenazine, Promethazine

b) Butyrophenone derivatives: Haloperidol, Droperidol

c) Other: Pimozide, Molindone, Doxapine, Risperidone, Clozapine, Quetiapine

2- Atypical:

a) Dibenzoxazepine: Loxapine

b) Dibenzoxazepine: Clozapine and olanzapinamolindone

c) Others: Sulpiride and risperidone

<u>- Psychostimulants:</u>

1- Convulsants and respiratory or analeptic stimulants.

2- Psychomotor or psychotonic stimulants (amphetamine, methylphenidate, caffeine, cocaine)

3- Psychotomimetics or psychedelics.

<u>- Antiepileptics:</u>

a) Voltage-dependent sodium channel inhibitors:

I) Prolong rapid inactivation: carbamazepine, eslicarbazepine, phenytoin, lamotrigine, oxcarbazepine and rufinamide.

II) Prolong slow inactivation: lacosamide.

b) Inhibitors of voltage-dependent broth channels:

I)   High voltage-activated P/Q channels: gabapentin and pregabalin.

II)   Low voltage-activated T channels: ethosuximide.

c) Potentiators of GABAergic tone:

I)   By blockade of the GAT-1 transporter: tiagabine.

II)   By GABA-transaminase inhibitor: vigabatrin.

III)   By activation of GABA receptors[A] : benzodiazepines, stiripentol and phenobarbital. d)AMPA receptor antagonists: perampanel.

e) Modulators of SV2A proteins of synaptic vesicles: leveriracetam and bribaracetam.

f) Antiepileptic drugs that act through multiple mechanisms of action: valproic acid, topiramate and zonisamide.

- Antiparkisonians:

1- Agents with prodopaminergic activity:

a) Levodopa

Levodopa associated with dopa-decarboxylase inhibitor: madopar and sinemet

b) Dopaminergic agonists: Bromocriptine, pergolide, lisuride, carbegoline.

c) Neuroprotectors: Amantadine

d) New dopaminergic agonists: Pramipexole, ropinirole, talipexole

e) Monoamine oxidase B enzyme inhibitors:Deprenil

f) Catechol-O-methyltransferase enzyme inhibitors: Tolcapone, entacapone

2- Agents with anticholinergic activity:

a) Muscarinic antagonists: biperidene, procyclidine, benztropine

b) Antihistamines with anticholinergic properties: diphenhydramine

c) Antidepressants: amitriptyline, imipramine, trazodone

Physiological changes of aging implicated in drug use.

<u>**Pharmacokinetic changes:**</u>

Pharmacokinetics refers to the processes to which drugs are subjected in the body: absorption, distribution, metabolism and excretion. Each of these is modified in different ways with the aging process.

Absorption:

In the older adult, gastric acid production, gastric emptying, gastrointestinal motility and blood flow as well as the absorption surface of the small intestine decrease, but the absorption of most drugs that pass through the gastrointestinal epithelium does not decrease, this being the pharmacokinetic parameter that is least affected. [29]

Distribution:

With age there are changes in body composition that affect distribution. These are:

Decrease in total body water by 10-15%: in addition to this there is a reduction in osmoreceptor sensitivity with less thirst sensation and favoring hypovolemic states. The decrease in body water means that water-soluble drugs have a lower volume of distribution and therefore reach their maximum plasma concentration more quickly and there is a greater risk of intoxication.

Increase and redistribution of body fat: there is an increase in abdominal fat, with less subcutaneous and limb fat. In addition, intramuscular and intermuscular fat deposits increase (myosteatosis). The increase in body fat causes fat-soluble drugs to have a greater volume of distribution and therefore a longer half-life, resulting in a delay in the onset of their maximum effect and accumulation with continued use. Examples of liposoluble drugs are diazepam, chlordiazepoxide.

The decrease in plasma albumin leads to an increase in the fraction of free drug in plasma with the consequent risk of toxicity. In addition, as polymedication is common in elderly patients, the reduction of drug binding capacity to albumin is particularly important, due to the displacement of albumin produced by other drug(s), with the consequent occurrence of adverse drug reactions (ADRs). For example, diazepam causes increased sedation.[29, 30]

Metabolism:

Aging brings with it a reduction in liver mass, hepatic blood flow (a decrease of 0.3-1.5% per year, and 40% at age 65) and hepatic metabolic capacity. The oxidation process (phase I reactions) decreases with age, and drugs using this system are biotransformed more slowly and tend to accumulate in the body. Benzodiazepines are metabolized by phase I reactions, except for lorazepam, oxazepam and temazepam; therefore, the latter are the drugs of choice in the elderly patient. Conjugation reactions (phase II) do not seem to be affected by age. [31]

Excretion:

In the elderly, renal changes occur that alter excretion, decreasing glomerular filtration (gradually by 35% between 20 and 90 years of age), tubular function and renal plasma flow. The elimination half-life of a large number of drugs increases, being necessary to take extreme precautions with the use of those that are nephrotoxic.[8, 28]

<u>Pharmacodynamic changes.</u>

Age-associated pharmacodynamic changes are often unpredictable and lead to failures in therapy, resulting in adverse drug reactions. These changes are less studied than pharmacokinetic changes and are only known for certain drugs.[29, 32, 33]

The biological aspects that alter drug behavior in the elderly are:

- Interindividual variability in response, and even within the same individual. May vary depending on the target organ. It is necessary to individualize the dose of each drug.

- Reduced capacity for internal homeostasis and external adaptation to changes. There is a slowing of complex responses that require coordination between different organ systems (water-electrolyte balance, glycemia, temperature, blood pressure) and therefore they are more sensitive to changes in thermoregulation produced by phenothiazines and anticholinergics.

- Increased sensitivity to drugs acting on the central nervous system (CNS). It is recommended to start with lower doses than those recommended in young people. Although sensitivity to benzodiazepines is increased, tolerance and dependence processes occur to the same extent as in young people.

- Decreased sensitivity of the thirst center and osmoreceptors, with the consequent tendency to dehydration. Therefore, the first and most effective therapeutic measure to be taken is hydration of the patient,

- Decrease in the number and affinity of specific receptors. The decrease in ^-receptor sensitivity may cause a lower intensity in the clinical response to ^-blockers and ^-agonists. This happens also with receptors to$_2$ -adrenergic receptors, while the sensitivity of a1-receptors does not seem to be affected.

- Changes in the cholinergic system. Not well known, it has been observed that the anticholinergic effects induced in the CNS, such as delirium and memory impairment, may be more pronounced in the elderly and produce RAM due to oversedation.

The anticholinergic effect is a strong predictor of disability and cognitive impairment, so drugs with this effect should be identified early to ensure maximum safety. Table 1 below summarizes some 34 psychotropic drugs according to anticholinergic risk scale.

Table 1. Anticholinergic risk scale.

1 point (low risk)	2 points (moderate risk)	3 points (high risk)
Amitriptyline Chlorpromazine Fluphenazine Hydroxyzine Hydroxyzine Imipramine Promethazine Tizanidine	Clozapine Nortriptyline Olanzapine Desipramine	Levodopa-Carbidopa Haloperidol Mirtazapine Quetiapine Trazodone Risperidone

Source: Salahudeen MS, Duffull SB, Nishtala PS. Anticholinergic burden quantified by anticholinergic risk scales and adverse outcomes in older people: a systematic review. BMC Geriatr. 2015, 31. Available at: https://doi.org/10.1186/s12877-015-0029-9

- The baroreceptor reflexes are less sensitive, becoming less effective and, therefore, the incidence of orthostatic hypotension due to the administration of any hypotensive drug is higher. This orthostatic hypotension is accentuated by drugs acting on the CNS (phenothiazines, tricyclic antidepressants (TCA), levodopa).

In addition to the physiological changes inherent to age, elderly patients often present associated multipathology, especially cardiovascular, metabolic, respiratory, renal and nervous diseases. These diseases and the treatments they require have a singular influence on the choice of the most appropriate psychotropic drugs for each patient.[35]

Actions of psychotropic drugs on some senile systems:

- Central nervous system:

Sedation:

It is necessary to consider the greater sensitivity of the elderly to the central depressant action of psychotropic drugs. For this reason, the sedative effects of most of them are increased. Sedation, which is different from anxiolysis, is an eventuality to be avoided as a general rule because of its impact on functionality and the increase of highly problematic events, such as falls. Both selective serotonin reuptake inhibitors (SSRIs) and dual inhibitors are characterized by their low sedative power compared to other existing antidepressants.[36]

Anticholinergic effects:

These effects are very relevant for certain psychotropic drugs and have a high impact on the functionality and quality of life of elderly patients. Central muscarinic blockade produces sedation, confusion and alteration of cognitive functions. This action causes cognitive impairment and aggravates pre-existing cognitive impairment if present. In the case of pre-existing cognitive impairment or dementia, it is particularly relevant and contraindicates the use of the most anticholinergic drugs, such as tricyclic antidepressants and certain neuroleptics. In the peripheral system, the anticholinergic action manifests itself mainly in the form of dry mucous membranes, constipation with risk of fecal impaction, decreased sweating, blurred vision, difficulty or retention of urine and tachycardia. Therefore, patients suffering from glaucoma, prostate hypertrophy, heart failure or diabetic gastropathy may suffer aggravation of their symptoms.[32,36]

Extrapyramidal effects:

Drugs with central dopaminergic activity can produce extrapyramidal symptoms or exacerbate pre-existing symptoms with important functional repercussions. It should be remembered that this effect does not only affect antipsychotics, since other drugs such as certain antidepressants can produce them.[36]

Epilepsy:

Elderly people with epileptic diseases should monitor their regular treatment with anticonvulsants in the case of concomitant use of many psychotropic drugs, since they can lower the seizure threshold as well as antipsychotics, especially conventional ones and clozapine. Atypicals and haloperidol have a lower risk.[35]

- *Cardiovascular system:*

Blood pressure:

Special attention should be paid to the vascular effects of drugs, since geriatric patients have greater lability due to baroreceptor degeneration. This fact leads to a higher incidence of orthostatic hypotension, which can precipitate syncope and falls. Because of their noradrenergic action, some drugs can, on the contrary, raise blood pressure. Tricyclic antidepressants usually produce orthostatic hypotension, which can be marked. Of these, nortriptyline is the least likely to cause hypotension, and is therefore useful in patients with congestive heart failure who need to take them. [36,37]

Cardiac conduction:

The cardiac conduction system is also more sensitive in the elderly and there is a greater risk of arrhythmogenic effects of certain drugs, some of which themselves lengthen the QT interval. Modern antidepressants exert minimal effects on cardiac conduction and have virtually no effect on ejection fraction. In contrast, the arrhythmogenic effect of ADTs is well documented and has been associated with an increase in sudden cardiovascular death, especially but not only in patients with ischemic heart disease. Contraindications extend to patients with acute coronary syndrome, recent infarction or conduction disturbances. For this reason, electrocardiographic monitoring of the patient should be performed after starting antidepressant treatment.[38]

Most atypical antipsychotics prolong ventricular repolarization, which is manifested on the electrocardiogram by an increase in the QT interval. The safest antipsychotics in these cases are haloperidol, risperidone, olanzapine and aripiprazole, which slightly increase the QT interval and do not cause ventricular arrhythmias.

However, administration of risperidone in geriatric patients with atrial fibrillation may increase thrombogenic activity.

Thioridazine, which have a lower risk of extrapyramidal symptoms, possibly due to increased antimuscarinic activity, but are rarely used due to problems related to QT prolongation and risk of polymorphic ventricular tachycardia.[32,38,39]

- *Endocrine system and metabolism:*

Carbohydrates and lipids:

It is necessary to monitor the appearance or worsening of problems related to glucose and lipid metabolism. Thus, certain molecules can cause a glucose imbalance, produce or aggravate diabetes (and interfere with antidiabetic treatment) or induce increases in cholesterol or triglycerides.

Weight:

The effects on appetite and weight are important in the elderly. Many of them are obese and should not be treated with medications that increase their weight. On the contrary, there are clinical situations that produce weight loss or constitutional syndrome that should be taken into account so that they are not aggravated by psychopharmacological treatment.

Hyperprolactinemia:

Increased prolactin has a clinical significance not yet well determined in the elderly, but it can produce or aggravate osteoporosis and cause sexual dysfunction. Osteoporosis affects a large part of the geriatric population and in cases of increased bone loss it is a condition to be taken into account when selecting drugs.

Hyponatremia:

Another factor to watch out for is the potential production of hyponatremia and syndrome of inadequate antidiuretic hormone secretion. Hyponatremia produces symptoms that can be mistaken for depression or dementia, such as bradypsychia, psychomotor slowing, emotional flattening, cognitive difficulties and confusion.[35,36]

- *Renal function:*

Patients with renal insufficiency, except in severe stages, do not often require very important dose adjustments of psychotropic drugs, since most of them are fat-soluble and do not depend exclusively on the kidney for their elimination.

Lithium and gabapentin, whose elimination is mainly renal, do require significant dose adjustments. The rest can generally be used safely in case of mild or moderate renal insufficiency.

Most psychotropic drugs, except lithium, gabapentin, pregabalin, valproic acid, risperidone and topiramate, cannot be eliminated by dialysis due to their large body volume of distribution due to their liposolubility and high binding to plasma proteins.[40,41]

- *Liver function:*

Most psychotropic drugs are metabolized and eliminated by the liver and in case of hepatic insufficiency their biotransformation and that of their metabolites is diminished, resulting in an increase in plasma concentration, with risk of toxicity. For this reason, elderly patients with liver disease will often require treatment adjustments. While acute hepatitis does not require changes in treatment, patients with chronic conditions - especially cirrhosis - will require a dose adjustment according to the degree of hepatic involvement. Of all the BZDs, loracepam and oxacepam, due to their intermediate half-life and lack of active metabolites, present less risk of accumulation and are therefore the safest BZDs in this situation. The use of long half-life BZDs is not recommended.[40,41,42]

Psychotropic drugs with lower risk profile according to medical pathology.

The following are the psychotropic drugs with the lowest risk profile (Table 2)

Table 2.Psychotropic drugs with lower risk profile according to medical pathology.

Psychotropic drugs	Types of medical pathology		
	Hepatic	Cardiac	Renal
Antidepressants	SSRIs (paroxetine, sertraline, escitalopram) SNRIs (desvenlafaxine)	SSRIs (escitalopram, sertraline)	SSRI
Antipsychotics	Haloperidol, sulpiride, amisulpride	Haloperidol	Haloperidol, olanzapine
Mood stabilizers	Lithium	V alproate, carbamazepine, lamotrigine, carbamazepine, lamotrigine	Valproate, carbamazepine, lamotrigine
Anxiolytics and Hypnotics	Lorazepam	Benzodiazepines, zolpidem, buspirone	Lorazepam, zopiclone

Source:Silva Hernán. Psychoarthropology and medical pathology. Clinica Las Condes
Medical Journal. 2017; 28(6); 830-4.
Available at: https://doi.Org/10.1016/j.rmclc.2017.09.002

Psychotropic drugs of choice in health problems associated with aging:

<u>Depression.</u>

According to the WHO expert committee on gerontosychology, depression is the most common health problem in the older adult population, conditioned by biological, psychological and sociocultural factors; it is also the most frequent geriatric syndrome in the outpatient clinic of patients over 60 years of age, causes a high degree of disability and represents a socio-family and public health problem. It is estimated that one out of every ten older adults suffers from it more or less periodically; and it is estimated that only one out of every three goes to the doctor and gets treated.[43]

Antidepressant therapy in the elderly is often complicated by comorbidity of diseases, polypharmacy and increased sensitivity to the effects of drugs. The following precepts are necessary for an adequate medication approach to depression in this group:[44]

- Use at the beginning half the doses as in the younger adult.
- Therapeutic doses should be achieved progressively.
- Be aware of the side reactions of the selected drug.
- Specify the medications taken by the patient.

The ideal antidepressant for use in older adults should not be cardiotoxic, lack orthostatic effects, have low sedative power, not interfere with memory and not cause functional alterations. Once the desired therapeutic response is obtained, maintenance treatment should be longer (not less than 1 year). Tricyclic antidepressants due to their anticholinergic effect (blurred vision, constipation, dry mouth, sinus tachycardia, urinary retention, mental confusion and delirium syndromes); cardiovascular (orthostatic hypotension, sinus tachycardia, antiarrhythmic effects and edema of lower limbs), are not recommended in older adults, and are also contraindicated in patients with cognitive disorders, in those with ischemic heart disease and orthostatic hypotension.

Selective serotonin reuptake inhibitors have fewer adverse effects than tricyclic antidepressants, with the exception of paroxetine which produces slight sedation and anticholinergic effects. These antidepressants provide safety, efficacy and reduction of unwanted effects, being the group of choice in the treatment of depression in the elderly. In addition to these drugs, other treatment alternatives can be used, such as occupational therapy, music therapy, play therapy, zootherapy and physical activity.[44,45]

<u>Insomnia.</u>

Sleep disorders are globally characterized by difficulty in sleep initiation and maintenance, and include:

a) Dyssomnia: these include intrinsic sleep disorders (psychophysiological insomnia and idiopathic insomnia), extrinsic sleep disorders (due to inadequate sleep hygiene, dependence on ethyl alcohol, psychostimulants and hallucinogens) and circadian rhythm-related sleep disturbances (travel across time zones, delayed or advanced sleep phase syndrome, or frequent shift work).

b) Parasomnias (sleepwalking, somniloquy and night terrors).

c) Sleep disorders associated with psychiatric conditions (schizophrenia, major depression, depressive dysthymia, chronic generalized anxiety, panic disorder, obsessive-compulsive disorder and post-traumatic stress syndrome),

d) Sleep disorders linked to neurological conditions (degenerative brain diseases, dementias, sleep onset epilepsy and nocturnal headache).[46,47]

Analysis of the classification of sleep disorders shows that a hypnotic drug is not indicated for all forms of insomnia. Thus, a significant improvement in insomnia associated with major depressive syndrome, schizophrenic syndrome or chronic generalized anxiety has been observed when the patient receives the specific medication (antidepressant, antipsychotic and anxiolytic) for that type of psychiatric condition. In addition, there are some forms of insomnia in which hypnotics are contraindicated. In clinical situations where hypnotics are indicated, treatment should be complemented by good sleep "hygiene" or "education" and behavioral therapies.[47]

The ideal hypnotic is a drug that shortens sleep latency rapidly and predictably, maintains sleep for a period of 7 to 8 hours, avoids frequent awakenings, preserves sleep architecture (maintains all stages of non-REM and REM sleep in their correct percentages). It does not generate immediate (morning hours) or late (weeks or months after starting treatment) adverse effects, does not produce abuse, tolerance or physical dependence after prolonged administration.

In transient insomnia, the administration of a hypnotic with a short mean elimination time may be necessary. Midazolam (7.5 mg), triazolam (0.125 mg for a period not exceeding 3 days) are indicated.

In short-term insomnia, a good sleep "hygiene" is particularly important (increasing physical activity during the evening hours, avoiding mentally stimulating situations, regularizing bedtime, avoiding naps, restricting the consumption of coffee, tea, cola drinks and alcohol, as well as heavy meals, and getting up at the same time in the morning), to which a hypnotic with a short average elimination time can be associated. The treatment will not be prolonged beyond 3 weeks.

In patients with long-term or chronic insomnia, a thorough medical-psychiatric evaluation is necessary. When a psychiatric condition is diagnosed, the administration of specific drugs (antidepressants, antipsychotics or anxiolytics) will result in an improvement of the clinical picture, including insomnia. If necessary, a hypnotic with a short elimination half-life may be associated. The situation is similar when there is a neurological condition (Alzheimer's disease, Parkinson's disease, epilepsy).[47,48]

<u>Parkinson's disease.</u>

Parkinson's disease is a complex neurodegenerative disorder that clinically presents with a combination of motor, autonomic and mental symptoms.[49]

The disease has heterogeneous subtypes according to presentation, response to medication and progression.[50] Most medications used to treat non-motor symptoms work through neurotransmitter systems other than dopamine. Treatments for non-motor symptoms are similar to those used in non-Parkinson's disease populations.[51]

For Parkinson's dementia, rivastigmine (3-12 mg/day) is clinically useful. Donepezil and galantamine are likely to be beneficial. There is no evidence to support the indication of memantine.[52]

Depression can be treated with pramipexole, tricyclic antidepressants (amitriptyline 12.5-75 mg/day or nortriptyline 5-50 mg/day in three doses per day), selective serotonin reuptake inhibitors (paroxetine 20-40 mg/day, mirtazapine 15-30 mg/day, sertraline 50-100 mg/day), or selective serotonin and noradrenaline reuptake inhibitors (venlafaxine extended release 37.5-150 mg/day or duloxetine 30-90 mg/day).[53,54]

Treatment of psychosis begins with withdrawal of potentially aggravating drugs (anticholinergics, amantadine, dopamine agonists, MAO-B inhibitors). Sometimes, discontinuation is limited by the reappearance of motor symptoms.

When psychosis persists and requires treatment, one of the following three options is preferred: 1) pimavanserin (third-generation atypical antipsychotic at a dose of 40 mg once daily), 2) clozapine (12.5-50 mg/day; with regular cardiological and hematological monitoring because of the risk of neutropenia), or 3) quetiapine (25-200 mg/day); this is the most convenient antipsychotic drug to prescribe.[55]

REM sleep behavior disorder is treated with melatonin (3-15 mg/day) as a first-line agent, but clonazepam (0.5-4 mg/day) may be necessary. Benzodiazepines may alleviate insomnia and anxiety, but worsen the function 56

cognitive.

<u>Epilepsy of the Elderly.</u>

Epilepsy in the elderly is that which begins in persons 60 years of age or older. It excludes those that begin at younger ages and remain in this age group. Isolated and recurrent epileptic seizures occur more frequently in the elderly because they are secondary to conditions that appear in these years.[57]

The treatment of epilepsies cannot be reduced to the simple administration of drugs and always requires taking into account the patient's global reality and, frequently, a multidisciplinary approach to the patient. For the acute management of the seizure, the airway should be kept patent, oxygen therapy if necessary, venous cannulation, and immediate medical treatment if necessary. Look for causes that require urgent treatment and prevent complications such as trauma or bronchial aspiration.

Most of the existing antiepileptic drugs (AEDs) show similar efficacy in treating the seizures that occur most frequently in the elderly (symptomatic focal epilepsies). In this context, the choice of drug will depend on its pharmacokinetic profile and the possible undesirable effects it may cause.

However, newer AEDs such as lamotrigine and gabapentin are more advantageous options than the older ones because they produce fewer undesirable neurotoxic effects.

Sodium valproate is also better tolerated in this population and produces fewer drug-drug interactions than carbamazepine and phenytoin. The elderly are especially susceptible to the sedative effect of phenobarbital and benzodiazepines which should be avoided.[58]

<u>Dementia.</u>

Dementia is not a specific disease. It is a general term that describes a wide range of symptoms associated with deterioration of memory and other thinking skills, which eventually reduce a person's ability to perform daily activities. <u>Alzheimer's disease</u> accounts for 60 to 80 percent of cases. Vascular dementia, which occurs after a stroke, is the second most common type of dementia. But there are many other conditions that can cause symptoms of dementia, including some that are irreversible, such as thyroid problems and vitamin deficiencies. [59]

While the symptoms of dementia vary widely, at least two of the following basic mental functions must be significantly affected to be considered dementia:[59]

- Memory

- Communication and language

- Ability to concentrate and pay attention

- Reasoning and judgment

- Visual perception

<u>Alzheimer's disease</u> is a degenerative disease characterized by progressive loss of cognitive function and altered behavior.[60]

Pharmacological treatment has four objectives: to delay deterioration, to maintain preserved functions, to recover some of the lost functions and to improve the patient's quality of life.

The main drugs used in its treatment are some acetylcholinesterase inhibitors (ACE inhibitors). At present, donepezil (10 mg/day), rivastigmine (6 to 12 mg/day) and galantamine (8 - 24 mg/day) are used. [61] **Self-medication with psychotropic drugs.**

One of the consequences of the current pace of life and the high demands to which society is exposed is the increase in chronic stress, as well as episodes of depression and anxiety. Associated with these social variables are other personal variables that aggravate these states, including a low tolerance to frustration or negative emotions, a poor approach to personal experiences or complex feelings.[62]

In today's society, one of the most common ways of coping with psychological distress in the face of many of these pressures is self-medication with psychotropic drugs.

Self-consumption of these drugs **is becoming more and more common**. Despite the fact that all of them are prescribed by a physician, many people resort to other means to have this resource to alleviate their discomfort, improve their night's rest or calm the anxiety that makes it difficult for them to manage their day-to-day life.[63]

The indiscriminate use of anxiolytics is undoubtedly the main problem when it comes to self-medication. Opting for this route without the prescription of a professional and with the appropriate psychological support, undoubtedly leads to a boomerang effect with very unfortunate consequences. **While it is true that at the beginning they can generate relief, little by little, the person will need higher doses to obtain the same effect**, ending up with a serious addiction. **In many cases, they can interact with other medications being taken,** increasing the risk of heart attacks and even death.[64]

The reasons why people resort to self-medication are multiple, most of them do so after having undergone medical treatment and feeling that their problem has not been solved, instead of seeking professional help once again, they opt for this route.

In another case, there are people whose relatives or friends are being treated with psychotropic drugs for a certain pathology and they **themselves identify with these symptoms and, without first having a medical consultation, decide to self-medicate.** This implies risks due to possible problems or events related to the drugs, which range from mild to serious, depending on the drug and the user. They can be toxic in cases of overdose, producing accidental, iatrogenic (adverse or unfavorable physical or mental condition) or intentional emergencies.[65]

The effects of self-medication with psychotropic drugs will depend on the type of medication the patient is taking. However, the most common is to experience the following:[62] - Drowsiness

- Muscle stiffness

- Tremors

- **Feeling of dejection**

- **Falls**

- Dry mouth

- **Constipation**

- Blurred vision

- **Heart problems, such as tachycardias**

- Allergic reactions

- Sexual dysfunction

- Restless legs syndrome

- Renal problems

Main adverse reactions of psychotropic drugs, according to pharmacological group.

Psycholeptics or CNS depressant drugs:

Some derive from the mechanism of action itself, while others are allergic in nature or of unknown causes; some appear immediately, at therapeutic doses or due to overdosage, while others are delayed.

I. Sedation and vegetative blockade

Sedation is completely independent of the neuroleptic action and does not contribute to the antipsychotic action; tolerance to the sedative action usually develops during the first few days.

II. Extrapyramidal reactions

Some are acute, due to overdosage: parkinsonism, dyskinetic movements and akathia; others appear in the course of chronic treatment: tardive dyskinesia. In acute cases, the phenomenon of tolerance appears. Neuroleptic malignant syndrome is a rare and serious reaction that appears with very high doses of potent neuroleptics. It is characterized by a state of catatonia, pulse and blood pressure instability, stupor, hyperthermia and sometimes myoglobinemia.

III. Cardiovascular reactions

Postural hypotension, secondary to a-adrenergic blockade, may cause nonspecific electrocardiographic alterations described above all in treatment with some phenothiazines, particularly thioridazine: prolongation of ventricular repolarization with QT space lengthening, widening, flattening or inversion of the T wave, bicuspid T wave and U wave.

IV. Allergic, dermal and pigmentary reactions

Phenothiazines, particularly chlorpromazine, may develop cholestatic jaundice of allergic nature. Agranulocytosis may occasionally occur, more frequently with clozapine, thioridazine and chlorpromazine. Allergic skin reactions in the form of photosensitivity are also observed.

V. Endocrine disorders

Weight gain, impotence, reduced libido, loss of ejaculation, gynecomastia with or without galactorrhea, amenorrhea and menstrual irregularities. Interactions

a. pharmacodynamic: they enhance the action of other central depressants: opioids, anxiolytics, hypnotics, anesthetics, anesthetics and alcohol

b. pharmacokinetic: due to their anticholinergic activity they can delay gastric emptying and the absorption of other drugs. Conversely, antacids can alter the absorption of neuroleptics. [66]

Anxiolytics or minor tranquilizers:

Benzodiazepines.

The most frequent are due to mismatch in relation to the desired effect. Sedation, drowsiness, ataxia, dysarthria, motor incoordination and inability to coordinate fine movements or to respond verbally or motorically to stimuli that require a quick response, alter the ability to drive vehicles. They can produce anterograde amnesia, that is, limited to events occurring after the injection.

More than to alterations in perception, it is due to alterations in the processes of consolidation and storage. Sometimes it can produce aggressive or hostile behavior, due to disinhibition, or an initial state of nervousness before the anxiolytic or sedative effect is established. With short-acting preparations, rebound anxious phenomena may appear when the drug's effect ceases.

Intravenously it can rapidly trigger hypotension and respiratory depression, but its lethal capacity is very small. The danger increases if associated with other CNS depressants: alcohol, anesthetics or opiates. Pharmacodynamic interactions are frequent when benzodiazepines are combined with other psychotropic drugs and are abused.

In relation to tolerance, it is produced to sedative and anticonvulsant effects, which is better appreciated when high doses are administered for a prolonged period of time. Tolerance is crossed with that of alcohol and other sedatives. They can also cause psychological and physical dependence, even at low doses, with a withdrawal syndrome that develops slowly after drug withdrawal. The symptomatology of the symptoms is such that in many cases it is difficult to differentiate whether it is a relapse of the original anxious condition or a withdrawal reaction. The higher the dose used and the longer the treatment, the more intense the symptoms are. The prescription of low doses and intermittent administration considerably minimizes the problem of tolerance and dependence.[11,67]

Hypnotics and sedatives:

Side effects observed during administration of benzodiazepine and non-benzodiazepine hypnotics include drowsiness and sedation, ataxia, dysarthria, diplopia, vertigo, dizziness, loss of recent memory, hostility reactions and depression. Most of these adverse effects can occur during the use of any of the hypnotics already described, but those of a depressant nature are more frequent when drugs with a prolonged elimination half-life are administered.[39]

Hypnotic tolerance

Tolerance to the hypnotic effect of benzodiazepines appears after the first or second month of treatment.

Insomnia rebound

Abrupt discontinuation of benzodiazepine hypnotics can lead to rebound insomnia. Insomnia rebound described for benzodiazepine hypnotics is characterized by the sudden and temporary reappearance of the symptoms for which the patient consulted, in an exacerbated form. During insomnia rebound, an increase in sleep onset latency, total wake time and wake time after sleep onset is observed. Total sleep time and sleep efficiency (ratio between the time the patient remains in bed and the time he/she sleeps) decrease; in addition, and due to frequent awakenings, sleep is very fragmented.[46]

Withdrawal syndrome

It may occur upon abrupt withdrawal of a benzodiazepine hypnotic that has been administered daily for weeks, months or years. The syndrome is characterized by the appearance of new symptoms of varying intensity and may persist, if untreated, for several weeks.

Withdrawal syndrome can occur: after treatment with therapeutic doses or, in dependent patients, with doses above therapeutic doses; after substitution of a hypnotic with a long elimination half-life for one with a short elimination half-life; after administration of a benzodiazepine antagonist. The symptoms observed during the withdrawal syndrome have been grouped into four categories:

a. Frequent and nonspecific: including sleep disorders, anxiety, dysphoria, irritability, muscle aches, tremor, headache, nausea, loss of appetite, weight loss, sweating and blurred vision.

b. Perceptual disorders of a quantitative nature: such as hypersensitivity to noise, light, odors, tactile and olfactory stimuli.

c. Disorders in the perceptual sphere of a qualitative nature: kinesthetic, optical, gustatory, acoustic and olfactory.

d. Heterogeneous symptoms: including depersonalization, psychosis and seizures.[47, 48]

Psychoanaleptic or stimulant drugs:

Tricyclic antidepressants:

Adverse effects of antidepressants can occur in up to 5% of patients. Several of them have potent actions on different central and peripheral receptors, from which many of the side effects of these drugs derive.

Antidepressants that selectively block serotonin reuptake show fewer adverse effects than the more classical ones. Among the most frequent are dry mouth, urinary retention, constipation, blurred vision, postural hypotension, palpitations, tachycardia, sedation and seizures.[68] MAO inhibitors:

They can produce hypertension, episodes of agitation and even hypomania and, very rarely, hallucinations and convulsions. In addition, other adverse effects have been reported such as diabetic neuropathy, dizziness, headaches, weakness, fatigue, dry mouth and constipation.[69]

Antimanic or mood stabilizers:

Lithium salts

When plasma lithium levels are higher than 1 mEq/l, intestinal disorders and anorexia usually occur. Above 1.5 mEq/l, muscle twitching, hyperreflexia, ataxia, somnolence, electroencephalographic alterations and even convulsions appear. These adverse effects are more probable in patients with renal insufficiency or patients on a sodium-free diet or undergoing treatment with diuretics that cause sodium depletion.[70]

Recommendations when prescribing to the elderly.

The following recommendations should be taken into account when prescribing to the elderly:[35]

- Obtain a complete medication history including allergies, adverse reactions, use of self-prescribed drugs, nutritional supplements, alternative medicine, alcohol, tobacco and caffeine use.

- Clearly assess and define the patient's problem. First consider the use of non-pharmacologic therapies before initiating a drug. Eliminate current drugs for which you cannot identify a clear reason for prescribing.

- Be aware of other diseases or other medications the patient is taking that may affect the choice of drugs. Medications may have an impact on pre-existing conditions or the action of other medications.

- Assign priorities to treatments, use as few drugs as possible.

- Use the lowest effective dose.

- To know the mechanisms of action, interactions, adverse events and toxicity profiles of the drug to be indicated.

- Continually evaluate whether the indicated therapy is effective and necessary.

- Monitor medication compliance.

- Consider the appearance of a new symptom as a possible adverse event.

- Encourage adherence to therapeutic recommendations. Educate the patient and caregiver about the medications. Provide written information, instructions and warnings in clear and understandable language.

- Avoid products in fixed combinations.

- Avoid the simultaneous use of more than one drug with similar actions.

In the elderly it is not just a matter of prescribing drugs, but of selecting the best, the most effective, but with the least adverse side reactions, in the lowest dose without deterioration of efficacy, using the most compatible pharmaceutical form, with the optimal intervals and adjusted to the biological requirements, but contemporizing with the psychological, emotional, social and economic eventualities of each aging individual, taking into account the potential benefits and risks for each patient. The high prevalence of psychiatric illnesses in primary care practices forces diagnostic and therapeutic decisions to be made, in many cases in haste. Assessing and diagnosing anxiety and depression problems in the short time available is a challenge and a clinical skill that is undoubtedly linked to the knowledge and experience of the family physician.[71]

Patient and family education.

It is necessary for the population to acquire basic knowledge on health issues, aimed at promoting healthy lifestyles (habits, customs, behaviors) based on the specific needs of the individual, family or community, with the objective of making health a collective good, training the population to contribute to their health in a participatory and responsible manner, changing harmful behaviors and consolidating healthy ones.

Informing the elderly, family members and caregivers about medications is a basic element that should be considered as another link in this process, which includes those aspects necessary for the success of pharmacological therapy.

When a patient needs to take a drug, he must have enough information to do it correctly. To do so, it is necessary for them to know the reason why they need to take the drug, the way it will act in their organism and the effect it will have on their disease. All these aspects help the patient to acquire a criterion on the benefit that the drug can bring to his health. In addition to these general aspects of the drug, it is necessary to tell the patient how to take it, what dosage and for how long, precautions to consider and/or adverse effects that may occur.

On learning all these details about the drug, the patient's attitude tends to be one of reinforcing his or her interest in following the treatment correctly, which is directly reflected in compliance. The main objective of the information process is to increase the patient's knowledge of the drugs, so as to facilitate their proper use, avoid undesirable effects as much as possible, and promote good compliance with the treatment.[72]

Design of actions.

Due to national projections and the growth of the elderly population, the demand for Geriatrics, Gerontology, Security and Social Assistance services is increasing. It is well known that the inadequate use of medications has serious consequences on the elderly and on the health system. In our country, according to studies, 81% of the elderly take medication.[25] Given their impact, different strategies have been proposed over time to optimize the use of drugs in these patients. The characterization of the geriatric population as being at high risk of mortality and disability - two essential indicators for the assessment of any therapeutic intervention - implies recognizing the importance of considering the elderly as a special group, especially for the analysis and evaluation of the effectiveness and safety of any medication.

Action planning consists of determining exactly what needs to be done to get where you want to go. It doesn't matter if it's about personal or organizational goals, as the skills needed are the same. The best strategies, both in life and at work, include action planning as part of strategic thinking.

After all, it doesn't matter how good the strategy is on paper if it can't be implemented. So action planning should be a crucial part of strategy. But it often isn't. To ensure that the organization is aligned, that is, that everything and everyone within it is aligned and working towards the organizational strategy, everyone in the organization must be able to explain and understand exactly how what they do fits into the overall strategy. This can only be achieved when the organization and the leaders are very clear about what actions will lead the organization to achieve its objectives.

Regarding the teaching-learning process with older adults, socialization is encouraged through a flexible and participative open education, promoting the integral development of the personality and allowing the development of capacities beyond the intellectual ones. The methodology recommended in this educational process is the application of group dynamics, not forgetting that these should be understood not as an end but as a means to achieve the objectives set.

The first phase in any planning process is to carry out a detailed analysis of the context in which the intervention will take place, in order to know the target group of the training action. The knowledge of the reality allows to carry out with more precision and efficiency the subsequent phases of the educational intervention.

Therefore, training actions with adults should be focused on the target group and aim at developing personal skills (self-knowledge, reasoning skills in decision making, problem solving), interpersonal skills (ability to accept group rules, work rules, self-discipline) and understanding and knowledge of different topics, work-related issues, leisure and relationships with people and family members. [73]

METHODOLOGICAL DESIGN

Type of study.

A descriptive observational cross-sectional study was carried out in older adults of the Medical Clinic N° 21 in the locality of Rodrigo, belonging to the health area of the Manuel Piti Fajardo Teaching Polyclinic of Santo Domingo, in 2021. It comprised two fundamental stages: one of diagnosis and the other of action design.

Universe and Sample:

Out of the total number of older adults dispensed who were consuming psychotropic drugs during the study period at the Medical Clinic N° 21, a sample of 53 was used.

Inclusion criteria:

- Voluntariness of the patient using psychotropic drugs by signing the informed consent form (Annex 1).

Exclusion criteria:

- Obvious mental incapacity to give consent and act accordingly to the study.

- Patients who emigrated from their place of residence before the period established for the study.

- Patient who was visited on more than three occasions by the investigator with prior notice and was not found.

- Patients living in an area located more than 3 kilometers from the Consultorio. Exit criteria:

- Voluntary abandonment.

- Death of the patient before completing the required information.

Procedure.

Initially, an interview (Annex 2) was conducted with each of the elderly by the researcher responsible for the study. A documentary analysis was also made (Annex 3). In the second stage of the study, based on the results obtained, a proposal of actions was prepared (Annex 4) to reduce the consumption of psychotropic drugs.

Operationalization of variables.

✓ Age: According to age at the time of the study.

Four ranges were established:

60 -69years

70-79years

80-89years

90 and over

✓ Sex: According to biological sex.

They were defined:

Female

Male

✓ Educational level: According to completed school grade referred by the patient in the interview and in the medical history review guide.

Four categories were established

Primary.

Basic secondary school.

Pre-university.

University

✓ Forms of use of psychotropic drugs:

Frequency of use: According to what was reported by the patient in the interview conducted during the research and information gathered in the medical history review guide, three categories were defined.

Sometimes: when the older adult consumes psychotropic drugs less than twice a week.

Almost always: when you use psychotropic drugs more than three times a week.
Always: when he/she uses psychotropic drugs on a daily basis.

Medication used: According to the information gathered in the guide for the review of the clinical history applied and what the patient referred to in the interview conducted during the investigation, two categories were defined.

Always the same: when the elderly person reported always using the same psychotropic drug.

The one that appears: when the elderly person reported using any psychotropic drug.

Amount of medication used: According to what the patient reported in the interview conducted during the research, two categories were defined.

Only one: when the patient reported using only one drug.

More than one: when the patient reported using more than one drug.

Type of psychotropic drug: According to Category and Pharmacological Action

- Antipsychotics
- Anxiolytics
- Hypnotics
- Antiparkisonians
- Anticonvulsants
- Antidepressants

Routes of acquisition: According to what the patient referred to in the interview and the information gathered in the medical history review guide, these were defined.

- Own route: when the elderly person reported acquiring psychotropic drugs without a prescription.
- Medical indication:

  - By their family physician: when the elderly person reported acquiring psychotropic drugs on the advice of their family physician.

  - By other specialists: when the elderly person referred to acquire the psychotropic drugs by indication of other specialists such as Psychiatrist, Neurologist or others.

<u>Reason for the use of psychotropic drugs</u>: According to the patient's statements in the interview, the following were defined.

- Sleep disorders: when the elderly person reported using psychotropic drugs due to a history of insomnia.

- Depression: when the elderly person reported using psychotropic drugs due to a history of depression.

- Anxiety: when the elderly person reported using psychotropic drugs due to a history of anxiety.

- Parkinson's disease: when the elderly person reported using psychotropic drugs because of a history of Parkinson's disease.

- Epilepsy: when the elderly person reported consuming psychotropic drugs due to a history of epilepsy.

- Other pathologies: when the elderly person reported using psychotropic drugs for any other illness, other than those previously stated.

<u>Occurrence of adverse drug event</u>: According to what was reported by the patient in the interview, two categories were established.

- If there was a suspicion of an adverse event derived from the consumption of drugs, understood as the appearance of any sign/s or symptom/s different from the one that motivated the consumption of the drug. That is not explained by the underlying disease and that is also in the profile of adverse effects of the drugs consumed.

- No: otherwise.

<u>Knowledge about the risks of psychotropic drug use in the elderly</u>: According to what was referred to by older adults and their caregivers in the interview (Annex 2), two categories were established:

- Knows: when the elderly person reported three or more risks.
- Don't know: when the elderly person reported less than three risks.

If the final result of the evaluation of the knowledge of older adults is that 60% or more are unaware, the proposal of actions is justified.

Ethical aspects.

The study was conducted under the criteria established in the Declaration of Helsinki (Ethical Principles for Medical Research Involving Human Subjects, adopted by the World Medical Assembly, Seoul 2008). It was adjusted to the norms established in the national and international codes of ethics and legal regulations in force in Cuba. The patient received the necessary information to decide to participate in the study. The research team explained the objectives of the study to each of the participants and obtained their informed consent (Annex 1). The information collected was only used for scientific and research purposes, without violating any of the established ethical principles.

Statistical analysis.

The results obtained were stored in the general Microsoft Excel database system to facilitate their analysis and processing using statistical software (SPSS), version 6 for Windows. In accordance with the type of study, statistical tables and graphs were prepared showing the absolute frequencies and percentage analysis of the data.

RESULTS

The distribution according to age group and sex showed that of the 53 older adults, 11 (20.8%) were male and 42 were female, the latter predominating with 79.2%. Within the male sex, the largest number of elderly was between 70 and 79 years of age (7, for 13.2%), followed by those between 60 and 69 (2, for 3.8%); and only one in the age groups between 80 and 89 and 90 and over. In the group of females, those aged 60 and 69 years predominated (19, for 35.8%) followed by those aged 70 and 79 (15, for 28.3%); and only 2 in the group aged 90 and over.(Table 1).

As for the distribution according to educational level, the largest number of seniors was at the pre-university level, 19 (35.8%), followed by elementary and junior high school with 13 (24.5%) and 11 (20.8%) respectively, and 10 university students (Table 2) (Table 2).

When analyzing the frequency of use of psychotropic drugs, it was found that 34 (64.1%) always used them, being the female sex the predominant one with 28 (52.8%), followed by those who almost always used them 10 (18.9%) and 9 (17.0%) used them sometimes; thus showing a high use of these drugs in the studied population (Table 3).

Of the total number of older adults, 15 (28.3%) reported always using the same drug, while 38 (71.7%) used the drug that appeared.(Table 4) When considering the amount of drug used, it was observed that 40 patients (75.5%) used more than one drug, represented by females with 28 (52.8%) and only 13 used the same drug, for 24.5%.(Table 5).

The most used pharmacological group in the study sample were hypnotics with a total of 42, with a predominance of 34 (64.2%) females and 8 (15.1%) males; within this group, Benzodiazepines were the most used. This was followed by anxiolytics with 19 (35.8%) in women and 5 (9.4%) in men. A lower use profile was found for anticonvulsants and antiparkisonics with 2 and 4 elderly people, respectively.(Table 6).

With respect to the routes of acquisition of psychotropic drugs in older adults (Table 7), it was found that 64.2% reported acquiring them by their own means, 24.5% corresponded to those who did so through other specialists and 11.3% through their family physician.

Table 8 shows the reason for the use of psychotropic drugs. A total of 52.8% reported sleep disorders, with a predominance of 39.6% of the female sex. This was followed by those who reported depression with 32.2% and Parkinson's disease and epilepsy with 4 each, for 7.5%.

When analyzing the occurrence of adverse drug events in older adults, it was found that 20.8% presented some manifestation, mostly due to dizziness, fatigue, gait incoordination and exacerbation of the symptoms for which the drugs were administered (Table 9) (Table 9).

When addressing the knowledge of older adults about the risks of psychotropic drug use (Table 10), it was found that 35 (66.1%) of the 53 patients were unaware of the risks, thus demonstrating that there is a poor command of the subject in question.

A proposal of actions (Annex 4) was designed to reduce the use of psychotropic drugs among older adults in the town of Rodrigo. Thirteen actions were conceived that independently responded to three main objectives. Group interviews, surveys and participant observation were proposed as forms of evaluation. Among the places suggested for the development of these actions were the Medical Clinic, the local House of Culture and the central park.

DISCUSSION

Current population aging is a global phenomenon without precedent in the history of mankind. The extension of life expectancy has been a longing throughout the years. In this sense, in our country, longevity can be considered an achievement to which the Cuban health system and primary health care, through the family doctor's plan where most of the care for the elderly is provided, have contributed a great deal.[74]

The current Cuban population shows demographic indicators of first world countries, low fertility levels since the late 80s of the twentieth century, low mortality levels, low and sustained values of infant mortality, coupled with a progressive growth in life expectancy at birth. A study[18] on population aging in Cuba shows that by the end of 2020, people aged 60 years and over doubled the figure of 1970, reflecting 21.3 percent of the total population, a figure that coincides with our study where when analyzing the province of Villa Clara we found that it is the most aged in the country, in the year 2021 25% of its population had or exceeded 60 years of age.[6]

Although there are no relevant findings, it is good to point out that the relationship between age and schooling of the patients studied was inversely proportional, the older the patient, the less schooling. It is not strange that in the younger age subgroup, higher levels of schooling were found if it is taken into account that these people have had better educational opportunities, similar results are found in a study on inappropriate use of psychotropic drugs in people aged 60 years and older in Cienfuegos.[22] In our study, 24.5% of the elderly had only completed primary school, with a predominance of middle and high school with 20.8% and 35.8% respectively, which was very useful for the understanding and operation of the proposed actions.

Mental health disorders in today's society make it a key area within primary care, not only because of the high prevalence of these disorders, but also because of the difficulty involved in their diagnosis, the high number of consultations it causes, the suffering it causes to patients and the consumption of psychotropic drugs involved. In our study we worked with elderly consumers of psychotropic drugs, it was observed that some of them consumed psychotropic drugs as part of the treatment of their chronic pathologies such as Parkinson's disease and epilepsy.

A large number of people need to acquire the product on which their well-being depends in the pharmacy network. These pharmacies are not sufficiently supplied to meet the demand, which leads the elderly to consume the drug they find to alleviate their symptoms, in our study most of them consumed the drug that appeared.

The endocrine-metabolic changes that occur in the female organism after menopause explain why many neurotic psychiatric disorders are more frequent in women and why the consumption of psychotropic drugs is higher. Benzodiazepines were the most commonly used in our research. A study carried out in the "30 de Noviembre" Community Polyclinic in Santiago de Cuba shows a predominance of the consumption of psychotropic drugs in women in the age group between 60 and 69 years, where the most consumed pharmacological group is Benzodiazepines[75] , coinciding with the results obtained by us.

There was a high percentage of consumption of psychotropic drugs by self-medication, the patients had access to them through non-conventional channels, not related to the health system and as for the reasons that led to their use, insomnia was the most frequent symptom corresponding to the most used drugs because BZD are indicated precisely for the treatment of sleep disorders. Similar results were found in a study of geriatric patients in a clinic in Venezuela, where insomnia and anxiety were the predominant symptoms.[76]

The effects of psychotropic drugs vary according to their chemical composition, the doses administered and the individual sensitivity of the patient.[31] The elderly are a high-risk group for adverse drug reactions due to the frequent association of multiple predisposing factors and a high degree of diagnostic suspicion should be maintained if several of them coexist: very advanced age, due to the pharmacokinetic and pharmacodynamic changes related to aging, with a longer half-life of the drugs and their plasma levels.[28,29] Pluripathology, especially if there are several intercurrent acute processes, highlighting renal and/or hepatic failure and metabolic alterations. Polypharmacy: this is the main risk factor for ADR.[36] The number of drugs taken: 5% if taking one to 100% if taking ten or more. The type of drugs, the doses used and the duration of treatment also play a role. Psychosocial factors: lack of social support can lead to poor compliance with treatment due to errors in taking and self-medication, especially if cognitive impairment, neurosensory deficit or poor manual dexterity are associated. Factors related to the prescribing physician: inadequate drug indications, excessive prescription with complex guidelines that are difficult to comply with and/or not correctly explained.[46]

The safety profile of a drug depends not only on its pharmacological profile (i.e. mechanism of action, pharmacological actions, interactions and pharmacokinetics), but especially on its proper use. The harm or risk of harm from any drug is obviously greater when it is used irrationally.

The study of adverse drug reactions is somewhat difficult since most of them are only reported when they require medical attention and many go unnoticed, creating an underreporting in this regard. In our study, the highest percentage of the older adults reported not having had adverse reactions, which disagrees with other studies where it is observed that these reactions are frequent.[62]

With respect to knowledge about the risks involved in the consumption of psychotropic drugs in the elderly, most of the elderly presented low knowledge, thus justifying the proposal of a system of actions.

Prescribing appropriately in the elderly is a difficult job that requires considering a balance between the risks and benefits of the indicated drugs, which usually do not have clear evidence of their efficacy, given the low representativeness of the elderly population in clinical trials, on which the clinical guidelines for the management of chronic diseases, conditions highly prevalent in the elderly population, are based.

We are faced with one of the most difficult problems to solve in the office on a daily basis. Patients are alone, without the company of their children, they are retired and, therefore, they perceive themselves to be out of the productive circuit. All these factors lead patients to tell us that they feel sad, anguished, discouraged and depressed, so that the prescription of psychotropic drugs increases to alarming figures without solving the main problem. On the other hand, self-medication reaches high levels in this regard, so it is essential to work to eliminate this behavior that, due to inappropriate doses and interactions with other pharmacological groups, affects older adults. We must therefore propose other therapeutic alternatives in which they can express their feelings and not "overshadow" them with the effect of drugs.

To this end, a series of actions are proposed in order to raise the awareness of this age group about the risks involved in consuming psychotropic drugs at this stage of life, linking community organizations in this work, in addition to the development of activities that allow the elderly to interact with each other, get out of the daily routine and stimulate skills that give them pleasure and improve their mental health.

CONCLUSIONS

In the population of older adults of the family medical office Nº 21 where high levels of consumption of psychotropic drugs are found, self-medication is a frequent practice and highlights the lack of knowledge of the risks involved in these behaviors in the elderly, actions are required to raise awareness, linking spaces and community projects to motivate this age group in a more enjoyable way. It is also necessary to increase their social relationships, seek new activities for their free time, build new relationships, have fun and feel more self-confident. All this allows the awareness of the elderly and the insertion of other alternatives that allow a better quality of life.

BIBLIOGRAPHIC REFERENCES

1. Alvarado García AM, Salazar Maya AM. Analysis of the concept of aging. Gerokomos [Internet]. 2014 Jun [cited 13 Jun 2022];25(2):[approx. 11 p.]. Disponible en: http//dx.doi.org/10.4321/s1134-928x2014000200002

2. Global index of aging, AgeWhatch 2015: executive summary [Internet]. [cited 2 Jul 2022]. Available from: http///www.globalagewatch.org

3. Granma P. Apply studies on population aging 170301: 2(1). 2017.

4. Amaro MC. Population aging in Cuba, from the prism of social epidemiology and ethics. Annals of the Cuban Academy of Sciences. 2016;6(2):30-45

5. Revuelta B, Acosta E. Aging and care in Cuba: The panorama and challenges of a "silent revolution". [Internet]. 2017 Mar 4 [cited 21 Jun 2022]:[approx.2p.]. Available from: http///www.cubaposible.com/envejecimiento- cuidados-cuba/.

6. Granma P. 25% of the population of Villa Clara is 60 years of age or older 100326: 2(1). 2021

7. García Chairez AL, Zegbe Domínguez JA, Ruíz de Chávez Ramírez D. Polypharmacy in the elderly in the first level of care. Semiannual electronic journal in Health Sciences. [Internet]. 2017 Dec 6 [cited 21 Jun 2022]:[approx.2p.].

   Available at: https://doi.org/10.48777/ibnsina.v8i2.35

8. Cala Calviño L, Dunán Cruz LK, Marín Álvarez T, Vuelta Pérez L. Main characteristics of drug prescription in elderly people at the "José Martí Pérez" Polyclinic. MEDISAN. 2017;21(12):3306-14.

9. Moreno-Martínez S, González-Hernández D, Hernández-Pizarro M, Concepción-Perdomo L. Consumption of antidepressants in the province of Artemisa in the period 2011-2017. Revista Cubana Farmacia [Internet]. 2020 [cited 3 Feb 2022]; 52 (4) Available from: https://revfarmacia.sld.cu/index.php/far/article/view/364

10. Gómez Mendoza C, León Martínez CA, Troya Gutiérrez Ag. Consumption of psychotropic drugs: a current health problem. Medicentro Electrónica [Internet]. 2020 Dec [cited 3 Feb 2022]; 24(4): 826-832. Available from: http://scielo .sld.cu/

scielo .php?script=sci arttext&pid=S 1029- 30432020000400826&lng=en. Epub 01-Oct-2020.

11. Rojas-Jara C, Calquin F, González J, Santander E, Vásquez M. Negative effects of benzodiazepine use in older adults: a brief review. Salud Soc.

[Internet]. 21 June 2019 [cited 3 February 2022];10(1):40-5. Available from: https://revistas.ucn.cl/index.php/saludysociedad/article/view/3611

12. Prevalence of psychotropic drug use in elderly population and observed side effects. Pilot study. Nuber Scientif. 2017;3(22): 22-28.

13. National Office of Statistics and Information. Cuba, 2016. [cited Diciembe 2022] Available from: http//www.one.cu

14. Sánchez Barrera O, Martínez Abreu J, Castel Florit S P, Gispert Abreu E, Vila Viera M. Population aging: some assessments from anthropology. Rev Méd Electrón [Internet]. 2019 May-Jun [cited: 20 January 2022];41(3). Available from: http://www.revmedicaelectronica.sld.cu/index.php/rme/article/view/3363/436

15. Boletin de Envejecimiento y Derechos de las Personas Mayores en América Latina y el Caribe. [Internet]. Dec 2021 [cited 3 February 2022]. Available from: http//www.cepal.org/es/notas/boletín-envejecimiento-derechos-personas-mayores

16. Ageism is a global problem-United Nations. Press Release. WHO. 18 March 2021. [Internet]. Dec 2021 [cited 3 Feb 2022]. Available from: https://www.who.int/es/news/item/18-03-2021-ageism-is-a-global- challenge

17. Statistical Yearbook. Latin America and the Caribbean. ECLAC; 2021. [cited March 2022] Available from: http://statistics.cepal.org/portal/cepalstat

18. The Aging of the Population. Cuba and its territories. 2020. July 2021 edition. [cited March 2022] Available from: https://www.onei.gob.cu/node/13821

19. Casanova Rodríguez CL, Cabrera EN, Cantero Tillet EI, Ramos Reyes IA. Factors associated with the health and well-being of the elderly. A case study in the province of Cienfuegos. Universidad y Sociedad [Internet]. 23 Apr 2019 [cited 3 Feb 2022];11(3):225-30. Available from:

https://rus .ucf.edu.cu/index.php/rus/article/view/

20. The misuse of prescription drugs- Research report. June 2020 [Internet]. 23 Apr 2019 [cited 3 Feb 2022] Available from: http://nida.nih.gov/es/publicaciones/los-medicamentos-de-prescripcion-abuso-y-addiction

21. Castro-Rodríguez JA, Marín-Medina D. Polypharmacy and prescription of potentially inappropriate medications in the elderly. Rev Med Risaralda. 2016; 22(1): 52-7.

22. Caro-Mantilla M, Apolinaire-Pennini J, González-Menéndez R. Inappropriate use of psychotropic drugs in people aged 60 years and older. Finlay Journal [Internet]. 2013 [cited 2022 Jan 24]; 3(1):[approx. 8 p.]. Available from: http://revfínlay.sld.cu/index.php/fínlay/article/view/174

23. Mental Health Atlas 2020. [Internet]. 2020 [cited 24 Jun 2022]. Available from: http://www.who.int/mental health/publications/mental-health-atlas-2020).

24. Lara-Bastanzur C, Calvo-Barbados D. Generalities of the Basic Drug List of Cuba in 2016. Cuban Journal of Pharmacy [Internet]. 2016 [cited 3 Jul 2022]; 50(2) Available from: https: //revfarmacia.sld.cu/index.php/far/article/view/19

25. Fernández Seco EA. Population aging in Cuba. Challenges of the health system. Conference. XV International Seminar on Longevity. April 2018. Havana: Palacio de Convenciones; 2018.

26. Coelho R, Veloso TM, Barros SM. Workshops with Mental Health Users: the Family as a Theme for Reflection. Psicol Cienc Prof [Internet]. 2017 [cited 25 Jul 2022]; 37(2): [approx. 10p.]. Available in: http://www.scielo.br/scielo.php?script=sci arttext&pid=S141498932017000200489&lng=en&nrm=i so

27. Torales J, Arce A. Principles of psychopharmacology: an introduction. Medicina Clinica y Social. 2017; 1(1): 54-99.

28. Flórez J, Pazos A. Central Nervous System. In: Flórez J, Armijo JA, Mediavilla A, editors. Human Pharmacology. Barcelona: Masson; 2014. p.407-568.

29. Rivera Paico ML, Vega Grados J. Characteristics of pharmacological prescription in hospitalized older adults at the Hospital Regional Docente las Mercedes Chiclayo, October 2016 - January 2017. Rev cuerpo méd HNAAA. 2017;10(2):69-74.

30. García Milián AJ. Drug Consumption and its Measurement. 2nd Edition. Havana: Ecimed; 2015.

31. Penny Montenegro E. Anatomic and physiologic changes during aging and their clinical impact. In: Melgar Cuellar F, Penny Montenegro E, editors. Geriatrics and gerontology for the internist. Bolivia: La Hoguera; 2012. p. 37-56.

32. Castillero Mimenza O. Types of psychotropic drugs: uses and side effects. Psychology and Mind. 2016; 20:21.

33. Oscanoa Espinoza TJ. Clinical pharmacology in geriatrics. 2nd Edition. Lima; 2012. p. 58-107.

34. Salahudeen MS, Duffull SB, Nishtala PS. Anticholinergic burden quantified by anticholinergic risk scales and adverse outcomes in older people: a systematic review. BMC Geriatr . 2015, 31. Available at: https://doi.org/10.1186/s12877-015-0029-9.

35. Pizarro Méndez D. Polymedication and inadequate prescription in older adults. Rev Médica de Costa Rica y Centroamérica. 2016;LXXIII(619): 389-94.

36. Angora-Cañego Ricardo, Esquinas-Requena José L, Agüera-Ortiz Luis F. Guide for the selection of psychotropic drugs in the elderly with concomitant medical pathology. Psicogeriatría. 2012;4(1):1-19

37. Salazar Cáceres PM, RottaRotta A, Otiniano Costa F. Hypertension in the elderly. Rev Med Hered. 2016;27:60-6.

38. Drugs that prolong the QT interval. Boletin Terapéutico Andaluz. 2017; 32(2)

39. Buxton IL, Benet LZ. Pharmacokinetics: dynamics of drug absorption, distribution, metabolism, and elimination. In: Brunton L, Chabner B, Knollman B, editors. The Pharmacological Basis of Therapeutics. Mexico: McGraw-Hill Interamericana; 2012. p. 17-40.

40. Ruíz A. **Psychopharmacology in special medical conditions. In:** Silva H, editor. Manual de Psicofarmacología Clínica. Santiago de Chile: Editorial Mediterráneo; 2016. p. 181 - 8.

41. Owen J, Crouse E. Pharmacokinetics, Pharmacodynamics, and principles of Drug-Drug Interactions. In: Levenson JL, Ferrando SJ, editors. Clinical Manual of Psychopharmacology in themedicallyill. Arlington: American Psychiatric Association Publishing; 2017. p. 3-44.

42. Silva Hernán. Psychopharmacology and medical pathology. Clinica Las Condes Medical Journal. 2017; 28(6): 830-4. Available at: https://doi.Org/10.1016/j.rmclc.2017.09.002

43. World Health Organization. Depression. Descriptive note. [Internet]. 2018 [cited 9 Jul 2022]. Available from: https://www.who.int/es/news-room/fact-sheets/detail/depression.

44. Perez R. Pharmacological treatment of depression: current events and future directions. Rev Fac Med [Internet]. 2017 [cited 9 Jul 2022];60(5):7-16. Available from: http://www.scielo.org.mx/scielo.php?script=sci arttext&pid=S0026-17422017000500007&lng=en

45. Quintana I, Velazco Y. Adverse reactions of antidepressants: current considerations. Rev Med Electron [Internet]. 2018 [cited 9 Jul 2022];40(2):420-32.

Available at: http://scielo.sld.cu/scielo.php?script=sci arttext&pid=S1684-18242018000200017&lng=en

46. Martínez Hernández O, Montalván Martínez O, Betancourt Izquierdo Y. Insomnia disorder. Current considerations. Rev Med Electron. 2019; 41(2).

47. D'Hyver de las Deses C. Sleep disturbances in older adults. Rev Fac Med Méx [Internet]. 2018 [cited 22 Jul 2022];(61):1. Available from: Available from: http://www.medigraphic.com/pdfs/facmed/un-2018/un181e.pdf

48. Aguilar Gómez B. Ramelteón: A drug for the fight against insomnia. Revista de Ciencias Universidad Pablo de Olavide [Internet]. 2018 [cited 23 Nov 2022]; (29):32-35. Available from:

https://dialnet.unirioja.es/servlet/articulo?codigo=6449717

49. Armstrong MJ, Okun MS. Diagnosis and Treatment of Parkinson Disease: A Review. JAMA. 2020;323(6):548-60.

50. Rodríguez García Pedro L. Diagnosis and medical treatment of Parkinson's disease. Cuban Journal of Neurology and Neurosurgery. 2020;10(1):e285.

51. Máñez JU, et al. Pilot study of a new tool to optimize dopaminergic treatment in Parkinson's disease: the OPTIMIPARK questionnaire. Journal of Neurology. [Internet]. 2021 [cited 15 Aug 2022] Available from: https://medes.com/publication/159323

52. Gomez LA. Cognitive impairment in patients with Parkinson's disease. Acta Médica del Centro. [Internet]. 2021 [cited 15 Aug 2022] Available from: http://revactamedicacentro. sld. cu/index.php/amc/article/view/1338.

53. Flores YG, Oliva JM. Factors associated with depression in older adults with Parkinson's disease treated in a Parkinson's workshop of the geriatrics service of the Naval Medical Center in 2018-2019. [Internet]. 2021 [cited 15 Aug 2022] Available from: https://repositorio.cientifica.edu.pe/handle/20.500.12805/1719

54. Torres MG, Ruiz YT. Depression in Parkinson's Disease in Older Adults.Millennial Knowledge. [Internet]. 2021 [cited 15 Aug 2021] Available from: https://cuazteca.edu.mx/revista/conocimiento%20milenario.pdf#page=51

55. Spanish Society of Neurology. Parkinson's disease. [Internet]. 2021 [cited 12 Jun 2021]: Available from: http://www.sen.es/114-videos/438-parkinson

56. Naranjo JE, et al. Sleep disorders in patients with Parkinson's disease. Cuban Journal of Neurology and Neurosurgery. [Internet]. 2021 [cited 15 Aug 2021] Available from: http://www.revneuro.sld.cu/index.php/neu/article/view/346/58

57. Millan Guerrero, RO; Isais Millan, R; Caballero Hoyos, R. Epilepsy in adults and the elderly in a Mexican population. Medicina Clinica Practica. 2022; 5(1):100.

58. Bombón-Albán PE. Pharmacological treatment of epilepsy in the elderly, review of the literature. Journal of Neuro-Psychiatry [Internet]. 21 Mar 2022 [cited 2 May 2022]; 85(1):55. Available from:

https://revistas.upch.edu.pe/index.php/RNP/article/view/4155

59. Custodio Nilton, Montesinos Rosa, Alarcón Jorge O. Historical evolution of the concept and current criteria for the diagnosis of dementia. Rev Neuropsychiatr. 2018; 81(4):235-50.

60. Cuba. National Center of Information on Medical Sciences. National Medical Library. Alzheimer's disease and other types of dementia. World Statistics. Factográfico salud [Internet]. 2021 Aug;7(8):[approx. 16 p.]. Available at: http://files.sld.cu/bmn/fíles/2021/08/factografico-de-salud-agosto-2021.pdf

61. Ministry of Health, Consumption and Social Welfare. Comprehensive Alzheimer's and other Dementias Plan (2019-2023): 41-44. Available at: http://www.mscbs.gob.es

62. Rodríguez López T, Salgueiro Labrador LS. Self-medication with psychotropic drugs in patients of medical offices in Pinar del Río. Rev Medical Sciences [Internet]. 2020 [cited 7 Jan 2022]; 24(1): e4020. Available from: http://revcmpinar.sld.cu/index.php/publicaciones/article/view/4020

63. Inter-American Drug Abuse Control Commission (CICAD), Organization of American States (OAS). Report on Drug Use in the Americas 2019. Washington, D.C.: CICAD, OAS; 2019.

64. Rodríguez ER, San Miguel Durand MÁ, Loya Espinoza W, Falcón Rodríguez D, Canelo Blas A. Level of self-medication of anxiolytics in users attending

apothecaries and pharmacies of the urbanization retablo del distrito de Comas. 2018. Lima: Universidad Interamericana; 2018.

65. Tobón Marulanda FA, Montoya Pavas S, Orrego Rodriguez MA. Family self-medication, a public health problem. Educ Med. 2018;19(S2):122-7.

66. Azón Belarre JC, Azón Belarre S, Pellicer García B, Berges Usán P, Abadía Labena S, Guajardo Iguaz A. Prevalence of psychotropic drug use in elderly population and observed side effects. Pilot study. Nuber Scientif. 2017;3(22): 22-8.

67. Gómez Saúl, León Tomás, Macuer Maximiliano, Alves Mariana, Ruiz Sergio. Benzodiazepine use in older adults in Latin America. Research Article. Rev Med Chile. 2017; 145:351-359.

68. Torres A. Tricyclic antidepressants: uses and side effects. A review of the functioning and positive and negative effects of this type of psychotropic drug. Psychology and Mind. 2021. Available at: https://psicologiaymente.com/login

69. Monoamine oxidase inhibitors (MAOIs). Learn about the risks, benefits, and side effects of these antidepressants. Mayo Clinic Sept. 12, 2019.

70. Malhi GS, Bell E, Outhered T, Berk M. Lithium therrapy and its interactions. Aust Prescr. 2020;43:91-3. Available at: https://doi.org/10.18773/austprescr.2020.024

71. Casas Vásquez P, Ortiz Saavedra P, Penny Montenegro E. Strategies to optimize pharmacological management in the elderly. Rev Peru Med Exp Public Health. 2016;33(2):335-41.

72. De La Guardia Gutiérrez MA, Ruvalcaba Ledezma JC. Health and its determinants, health promotion and health education. 2020; 5(1): 81-90.

73. García Rizo J. System of actions for the incorporation of the older adult to the Grandparents' Circles of the Eastern Popular Council, Morón Municipality. Digital Journal - Buenos Aires. 2013. Available at:

https://www.efdeportes.com>efd158

74. Romero Cabrera J. Clinical Assistance to the Elderly. 2nd Edition. Havana: Ecimed; 2012. p. 26-135.

75. Verdaguer Pérez L, Machín Rodriguez VT, Montoya Deler MA, Borrero Gorgas L. Consumption of psychotropic drugs in older adults in a health area. Acta méd centro [Internet]. 2021 Dec [cited 2022 Nov 04] ; 15(4): 521-30. Available from: http://scielo.sld.cu/scielo.php?script=sci_arttext&pid=S2709-79272021000400521&lng=en. Epub 31-Dec-2021.

76. Albear Caró F, Albear Caró Z, Hernández Creagh D. Consumption of psychotropic drugs in geriatric patients in a clinic in Venezuela. Rev Inf Cient [Internet]. 2015 [cited 26 Jun 2019]; 94(6):[approx. 8 p.]. Available from:

http://revinfcientifíca. sld.cu/index.php/ric/article/view/153/1197

ANNEXES

Appendix 1. CONSENT TO PARTICIPATE IN RESEARCH.

Study title: **Propuesta de acciones para disminuir el consumo de Psicofármacos en Adultos Mayores del Consultorio N 21. Rodrigo, 2021.**

I, Doctor Dailyn Lopez Santana, working at the Family Medical Clinic #21 in the town of Rodrigo, am conducting a research study on the use of psychotropic drugs in older adults. I hereby inform you that if you agree to participate, you will not suffer any harm to your health, you may abandon the study and it will not affect your subsequent health care. You will be interviewed, you will be visited at home and you must attend the doctor's office with a certain frequency, which you will be informed of at a later date. If you have any questions about it or your rights, please do not hesitate to ask before making your decision.

Me, ____

(Patient's first and last name written in his/her own handwriting)

o I have asked as many questions as I thought appropriate about the study.

o I have received satisfactory answers to my questions or doubts.

o I have received sufficient information about the study and understood it.

o I have spoken to ____

(Name and Surname of the clinical investigator, written in the patient's own handwriting)

o I understand that my participation is voluntary.

o I understand that I will not suffer damage to my health.

o I understand that I can withdraw from the study and this will not affect my attention afterwards.

o I freely agree to participate in the study and I will receive a copy of this document.

And for the record, I sign this consent along with the physician who gave me the explanations.

_______________________ |__|__|__|/|__|__|__|/|__|__| |__|__|:|__|__|__| □AM

□PM

Patient's Signature Date (day/month/year) **Time**

_______________________ |__|__|__|/|__|__|__|/|__|__| |__|__|:|__|__|__| □AM

□PM

Patient's Signature Date (day/month/year) **Time**

Annex 2. INTERVIEW WITH THE OLDER ADULT.

The purpose of this interview is to identify the main psychotropic drugs consumed by older adults in the health area, the reasons and ways in which they are acquired, as well as the knowledge they have about their use and the main adverse reactions associated with them. Please answer the questions honestly. The information collected will only be used for scientific, research and educational purposes. Your identity will be preserved and we will respect your decision not to cooperate with the research, if you wish to do so.

Data of interest:

Age: _________

Sex: ☐ Female ☐ Male

Level of education

If you are a Worker or Retiree

Whether you live alone or in company

Do you take any medication (psychotropic drugs). If yes, which one(s) Reason(s) for taking them

By whom they were indicated

Who supplies your medications

Frequency of use

---- Sometimes

---- Almost always

---- Always

Take only one psychotropic drug or more than one together.

Always use the same drug

Do you experience any symptoms or discomfort when taking these medications? If yes, which ones?

These unwanted effects disappear without treatment or other action.

If you ever feel well, do you stop taking the medication? Yes __ No __ No

Do you know about the risks of psychotropic drug use in older adults? If yes, give examples.

Yes you know: more than three

Do not know: less than three

Annex 3. REVIEW GUIDE

<u>The individual medical history and the Family Health Record will be obtained from the individual medical history and the Family Health Record:</u>

Chronic illness (history of psychiatric disorders)

Consumption of psychotropic drugs

Frequency of consumption indication

Educational level

Age

If you are a worker or retiree

Annex 4. PROPOSAL FOR ACTIONS TO REDUCE THE CONSUMPTION OF PSYCHOTROPIC DRUGS IN

OLDER ADULTS.

Based on the diagnosis of the current state of consumption of psychotropic drugs in the elderly, in the older adults of the Family Doctor's Office No. 21 in the town of Rodrigo, the need to propose actions to promote the adequate consumption of psychotropic drugs is evident.

General Objective:

To propose a system of actions to reduce the consumption of psychotropic drugs in older adults at the Family Medical Clinic No. 21 in the town of Rodrigo.

Specific objectives:

1- Promote awareness of psychotropic drug use and its risks in the elderly, in older adults.

2- Insert community projects in the town of Rodrigo as spaces for promoting the risks of psychotropic drug use among older adults.

3- To develop spaces for exchange and recreation that encourage social integration and improve physical and mental health among older adults.

Specific objectives	Shares	Location	Responsible party(ies)	Participants	Time (periodization)	Form of evaluation
Promote awareness of psychotropic drug use and its risks in the elderly, in older adults.	Exchange with residents and MGI Specialists trained in the subject of Psychotropic drugs.	Office Physician	Family Physicians	Older adults	Semiannual	Group interview
	To set up a Circle of interest in topics to be discussed on psychotropic drugs and their use in the elderly.	Local Cultural Center	Family Physicians	Older adults	Monthly	Participant observation
	Encourage discussions on "the risks of drug consumption psychotropic drugs".	Local Cultural Center	Family Physicians	Older adults	Semiannual	Survey
	Create spaces for counseling on ways of coping with the symptoms that lead to the use of psychotropic drugs.	Medical Office	Family Physicians	Older adults	Pennanente	Interview
	Exhibit and discuss audiovisual materials associated with the topic.	Local Cultural Center	Family Physicians	Older adults	Quarterly	Survey and participant observation

Insert community projects in the town of Rodrigo as spaces for promoting the risks of psychotropic drug use among older adults.	Disseminate issues, dates and research related to the promotion of the risks of psychotropic drug use in older adults.	Central Park	Teachers from the Institute of Sports and Recreation	Older adults	Pennanente	Survey
	To call for the production of a play that relates to the topic of psychotropic drug use in older adults and their main adverse reactions.	Local cultural center	Instructo res de Arte y Médicos de Familia.	Older adults	Annual	Participant observation
	Celebrate anniversaries related to the theme of the elderly (e.g., World Day of the Elderly, World Mental Health Day, etc.).	Central Park	Family physicians, older adults and their caregivers.	Older adults	Permanent	Interview

To develop spaces for exchange and recreation that encourage social integration and improve physical and mental health among older adults.	Create workshops for participation in the production of handicrafts and handicrafts.	House of culture.	Instructo res de Arte	Older adults	Permanent	Survey
	Organize a dance therapy circle.	House of Culture	Instructo res de Arte	Older adults	Permanent	Survey
	Promote spaces for planting medicinal plants.	Family Medical Office Orchard	Physicians and Family Nurse Practitioners	Older adults	Permanent	Participant observation
	Organize workshops for the elaboration of medicinal preparations from plants (infusions, decoctions).	House of Culture	Head teacher of the grandparents' circle in the community	Older adults	Semiannual	Survey and participant observation
	Conduct workshops on properties and ways of using medicinal plants that can substitute psychotropic drugs.	Casa de Adulto Mayor	Physicians and Family Nurse Practitioners	Older adults	Monthly	Survey and participant observation

TABLES

Table 1. Distribution of older adults according to age group and sex. Office Médico de Familia Nº 21. Rodrigo, 2021.

Age Group	Sex				Total	
	F		M			
	No	%	No	%	No	%
60 a 69	19	35,8	2	3,8	**21**	**39,6**
70 a 79	15	28,3	7	13,2	**22**	**41,5**
80 a 89	6	11,3	1	1,9	**7**	**13,2**
90 and over	2	3,8	1	1,9	**3**	**5,7**
Total	**42**	**79,2**	**11**	**20,8**	**53**	**100**

Table 2. Educational level of older adults according to sex. Medical Office of Family № 21. Rodrigo, 2021.

Educational Level	Sex				Total	
	F		M			
	No	%	No	%	No	%
Primary	12	22,6	1	1,9	13	24,5
Secondary	10	18,9	1	1,9	11	20,8
Pre-university	12	22,6	7	13,2	19	35,8
University	8	15,1	2	3,8	10	18,9
Total	42	79,2	11	20,8	53	100

Table 3. Frequency of use of psychotropic drugs according to sex. Medical Office of Family Nº 21. Rodrigo, 2021....

Frequency of use	Sex				Total	
	F		M			
	No	%	No	%	No	%
Almost always	8	15,1	2	3,8	10	18,9
Sometimes	6	11,3	3	5,7	9	17,0
Always	28	52,8	6	11,3	34	64,1
Total	42	79,2	11	20,8	53	100

Table 4. Medications used. Consultorio Médico de Familia Nº 21. Rodrigo. 2021.

Medication used	Sex				Total	
	F		M			
	No	%	No	%	No	%
Always the same	12	22,6	3	5,7	15	28,3
The one that appears	30	56,6	8	15,1	38	71,7
Total	42	79,2	11	20,8	53	100

Table 5. Quantity of medication used. Consultorio Médico de Familia Nº 21. Rodrigo. 2021.

Amount of medication	Sex				Total	
	F		M			
	No	%	No	%	No	%
Only one	7	13,2	6	11,3	13	24,5
More than one	28	52,8	12	22,6	40	75,5
Total	35	66	18	34,0	53	100

Table 6. Type of psychotropic drug used. Consultorio Médico de Familia Nº 21. Rodrigo. 2021.

Pharmacological group	SEX				TOTAL	
	F		M			
	No	%	No	%	No	%
Antipsychotics	4	7,5	0	0	4	7,5
Anxiolytics	19	35,8	5	9,4	24	45,3
Hypnotics	34	64,2	8	15,1	42	79,2
Antiparkisonians	3	5,7	1	1,9	4	7,5
Antic onvulsants	2	3,8	0	0,0	2	3,8
Antidepressants	21	39,6	5	9,4	26	49,1
Antimaniacs	1	1,9	0	0,0	1	1,9
Psychostimulants	0	0,0	1	1,9	1	1,9

Table 7. Acquisition routes. Consultorio Médico de Familia No 21. Rodrigo. 2021.

Acquisition channels		Number	%
Own way		34	64,2
Indication medical	By your family physician	6	11,3
	By other specialists	13	24,5

Table 8. Reason for the use of psychotropic drugs. Consultorio Médico de Familia Nº 21.
Rodrigo. 2021.

Reason for consumption	Sex				Total	
	F		M			
	No	%	No	%	No	%
Disorders of the dream	21	39,6	7	13,2	28	52,8
Depression	14	26,4	3	5,7	17	32,1
Epilepsy	3	5,6	1	1,8	4	15,1
Parkinson	2	3.7	2	3.7	4	7.5

Table 9. Occurrence of adverse drug events. Medical Office of
Family Nº 21. Rodrigo. 2021.

Adverse event	Sex				Total	
	F		M			
	No	%	No	%	No	%
Yes	8	15,1	3	5,7	11	20,8
No	34	64,1	8	15,1	42	79,2
Total	42	79,2	11	20,8	53	100

Table 10. Knowledge of older adults about the risks of drug use among older adults psychotropic drugs in the elderly. Consultorio Médico de Familia Nº 21. Rodrigo. 2021.

Knowledge	Number	%
Meet	18	33,9
Not known	35	66,1
Total	53	100

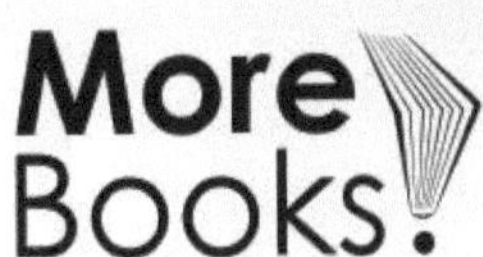

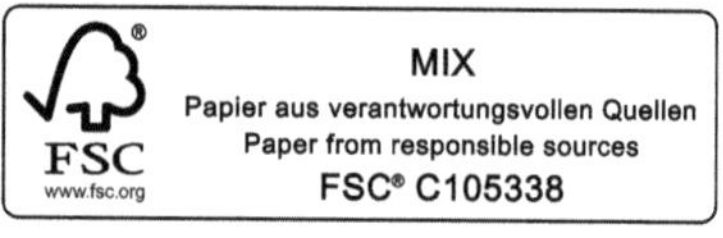

Printed by Books on Demand GmbH, Norderstedt / Germany